Seize the Day

Seize the Day

Matthew Petchinsky

Seize the Day: A Personal Seizure Tracking Journal
By: Matthew Petchisnky

Introduction to "Seize the Day: A Personal Seizure Tracking Journal"

Living with epilepsy or a seizure disorder can feel like navigating an unpredictable storm. Seizures can affect daily routines, physical health, mental well-being, and overall quality of life. Yet, understanding and managing seizures can lead to a sense of control and empowerment. "Seize the Day: A Personal Seizure Tracking Journal" is designed to be your companion on this journey—a place to document, reflect, and find patterns in your experiences, helping you and your healthcare providers make informed decisions.

The Power of Tracking

Why track seizures? Monitoring your seizures is one of the most effective ways to gain insight into their patterns and potential triggers. Keeping a detailed record helps identify factors that may provoke seizures, such as lack of sleep, stress, diet, hormonal changes, medication inconsistencies, or environmental factors. Over time, these patterns can reveal crucial information about how your body responds to different circumstances, making it easier to anticipate and manage future episodes.

Moreover, documenting your seizures provides valuable information for healthcare providers. This journal serves as a comprehensive record of your experiences, offering details that can guide treatment plans, medication adjustments, and lifestyle changes tailored to your unique situation. Sharing this information with your neurologist or epilepsy specialist allows for more personalized care, potentially reducing seizure frequency or severity.

How to Use This Journal

"Seize the Day: A Personal Seizure Tracking Journal" is thoughtfully structured to cater to your tracking needs. The journal is divided into daily, weekly, and monthly sections, making it simple to capture immediate details while also facilitating a broader overview. Here's how to make the most out of each section:

1. **Daily Logs** – These are at the heart of your tracking routine. Each day, you have a dedicated space to document seizure occurrences, including the time, duration, type, and potential triggers. It's also crucial to note any pre-seizure warning signs, commonly known as "auras," as well as how you felt afterward. Additionally, recording your medication intake, sleep patterns, diet, and stress levels can provide clues about factors that may be influencing your seizures. The daily log is designed to be straightforward yet comprehensive, allowing you to capture essential information without feeling overwhelmed.

2. **Weekly Summaries** – At the end of each week, you can step back and look for patterns or changes. The weekly log offers a space to tally the total number of seizures, review common triggers, assess medication adherence, and note any side effects. Reflecting on your experiences weekly can reveal trends that might not be immediately apparent day-to-day, helping you to adapt your lifestyle and treatment approach as needed.

3. **Monthly Overviews** – The monthly summary section is a powerful tool for identifying long-term trends. It allows you to document the total number of seizures, most common triggers, and the time of day seizures frequently occur. You can also review your medication regimen's effectiveness and jot down questions or concerns to discuss with your healthcare provider. These monthly reflections are invaluable for ongoing medical consultations, as they offer a consolidated view of your experiences and progress over time.

Benefits of Keeping This Journal

A seizure journal is more than just a record; it's a tool for empowerment. By actively tracking your seizures, you can work toward a better understanding of your condition. Here's how this journal can benefit you:

- **Increased Awareness**: Logging your seizures helps you become more attuned to your body's signals, making it easier to identify potential warning signs or patterns.
- **Improved Communication**: A well-kept journal provides concrete data for discussions with your doctor, leading to more informed decisions about treatment and lifestyle adjustments.
- **Enhanced Coping Strategies**: Identifying triggers and trends enables you to take proactive steps in managing your condition, whether it involves avoiding certain activities, adjusting sleep schedules, or working with your healthcare provider to explore new treatment options.
- **Emotional Support**: Writing about your experiences can be a therapeutic way to express your feelings, fears, and hopes. It also serves as a reminder of your strength and resilience as you navigate your unique path.

Your Journey to Better Understanding

"Seize the Day: A Personal Seizure Tracking Journal" is your personal space, meant to adapt to your journey. While it provides a structured format, there's room for flexibility—you can add notes, thoughts, or even sketches that capture your experiences in a way that feels meaningful to you. This journal isn't just about documenting seizures; it's about gaining insights, taking control, and empowering yourself in the face of unpredictability.

As you begin this tracking journey, remember that every detail you log brings you one step closer to understanding and managing your condition. Seizure tracking is an ongoing process, and your persistence will help uncover patterns that can make a real difference in your daily life. So, seize the day, capture your experiences, and take charge of your health with confidence.

Day 1

- **Date:** ____________
- **Time of Seizure:** ____________
- **Duration:** ____________ (e.g., seconds/minutes)
- **Type of Seizure:** ____________ (e.g., focal, generalized, etc.)
- **Triggers (if known):** ____________ (e.g., stress, sleep, flashing lights)
- **Warning Signs (Aura):** ____________ (e.g., dizziness, visual changes)
- **Description:**

What Happened:

After Effects:

Medication Taken (before/after):

Notes:

Day 2

- **Date:** ___________
- **Time of Seizure:** ___________
- **Duration:** ___________ (e.g., seconds/minutes)
- **Type of Seizure:** ___________ (e.g., focal, generalized, etc.)
- **Triggers (if known):** ___________ (e.g., stress, sleep, flashing lights)
- **Warning Signs (Aura):** ___________ (e.g., dizziness, visual changes)
- **Description:**

What Happened:

After Effects:

Medication Taken (before/after):

Notes:

Day 3

- **Date:** ___________
- **Time of Seizure:** ___________
- **Duration:** ___________ (e.g., seconds/minutes)
- **Type of Seizure:** ___________ (e.g., focal, generalized, etc.)
- **Triggers (if known):** ___________ (e.g., stress, sleep, flashing lights)
- **Warning Signs (Aura):** ___________ (e.g., dizziness, visual changes)
- **Description:**

What Happened:

After Effects:

Medication Taken (before/after):

Notes:

Day 4

- **Date:** ___________
- **Time of Seizure:** ___________
- **Duration:** ___________ (e.g., seconds/minutes)
- **Type of Seizure:** ___________ (e.g., focal, generalized, etc.)
- **Triggers (if known):** ___________ (e.g., stress, sleep, flashing lights)
- **Warning Signs (Aura):** ___________ (e.g., dizziness, visual changes)
- **Description:**

What Happened:

After Effects:

Medication Taken (before/after):

Notes:

Day 5

- **Date:** ___________
- **Time of Seizure:** ___________
- **Duration:** ___________ (e.g., seconds/minutes)
- **Type of Seizure:** ___________ (e.g., focal, generalized, etc.)
- **Triggers (if known):** ___________ (e.g., stress, sleep, flashing lights)
- **Warning Signs (Aura):** ___________ (e.g., dizziness, visual changes)
- **Description:**

What Happened:

After Effects:

Medication Taken (before/after):

Notes:

Day 6

- **Date:** __________
- **Time of Seizure:** __________
- **Duration:** __________ (e.g., seconds/minutes)
- **Type of Seizure:** __________ (e.g., focal, generalized, etc.)
- **Triggers (if known):** __________ (e.g., stress, sleep, flashing lights)
- **Warning Signs (Aura):** __________ (e.g., dizziness, visual changes)
- **Description:**

What Happened:

After Effects:

Medication Taken (before/after):

Notes:

Day 7

- **Date:** ___________
- **Time of Seizure:** ___________
- **Duration:** ___________ (e.g., seconds/minutes)
- **Type of Seizure:** ___________ (e.g., focal, generalized, etc.)
- **Triggers (if known):** ___________ (e.g., stress, sleep, flashing lights)
- **Warning Signs (Aura):** ___________ (e.g., dizziness, visual changes)
- **Description:**

What Happened:

After Effects:

Medication Taken (before/after):

Notes:

WEEK 1 REVIEW
Week Starting: ______________

• **Number of Seizures:** ______________

Patterns Noticed:

Common Triggers:

• **Medication Adherence: Yes / No**

Side Effects:

Notes for Healthcare Provider:

Day 8

- **Date:** _____________
- **Time of Seizure:** _____________
- **Duration:** _____________ (e.g., seconds/minutes)
- **Type of Seizure:** _____________ (e.g., focal, generalized, etc.)
- **Triggers (if known):** _____________ (e.g., stress, sleep, flashing lights)
- **Warning Signs (Aura):** _____________ (e.g., dizziness, visual changes)
- **Description:**

What Happened:

After Effects:

Medication Taken (before/after):

Notes:

Day 9

- **Date:** ___________
- **Time of Seizure:** ___________
- **Duration:** ___________ (e.g., seconds/minutes)
- **Type of Seizure:** ___________ (e.g., focal, generalized, etc.)
- **Triggers (if known):** ___________ (e.g., stress, sleep, flashing lights)
- **Warning Signs (Aura):** ___________ (e.g., dizziness, visual changes)
- **Description:**

What Happened:

After Effects:

Medication Taken (before/after):

Notes:

Day 10

- **Date:** ___________
- **Time of Seizure:** ___________
- **Duration:** ___________ (e.g., seconds/minutes)
- **Type of Seizure:** ___________ (e.g., focal, generalized, etc.)
- **Triggers (if known):** ___________ (e.g., stress, sleep, flashing lights)
- **Warning Signs (Aura):** ___________ (e.g., dizziness, visual changes)
- **Description:**

What Happened:

After Effects:

Medication Taken (before/after):

Notes:

Day 11

- **Date:** ___________
- **Time of Seizure:** ___________
- **Duration:** ___________ (e.g., seconds/minutes)
- **Type of Seizure:** ___________ (e.g., focal, generalized, etc.)
- **Triggers (if known):** ___________ (e.g., stress, sleep, flashing lights)
- **Warning Signs (Aura):** ___________ (e.g., dizziness, visual changes)
- **Description:**

What Happened:

After Effects:

Medication Taken (before/after):

Notes:

Day 12

- **Date:** ___________
- **Time of Seizure:** ___________
- **Duration:** ___________ (e.g., seconds/minutes)
- **Type of Seizure:** ___________ (e.g., focal, generalized, etc.)
- **Triggers (if known):** ___________ (e.g., stress, sleep, flashing lights)
- **Warning Signs (Aura):** ___________ (e.g., dizziness, visual changes)
- **Description:**

What Happened:

After Effects:

Medication Taken (before/after):

Notes:

Day 13

- **Date:** _____________
- **Time of Seizure:** _____________
- **Duration:** _____________ (e.g., seconds/minutes)
- **Type of Seizure:** _____________ (e.g., focal, generalized, etc.)
- **Triggers (if known):** _____________ (e.g., stress, sleep, flashing lights)
- **Warning Signs (Aura):** _____________ (e.g., dizziness, visual changes)
- **Description:**

What Happened:

After Effects:

Medication Taken (before/after):

Notes:

Day 14

- **Date:** ___________
- **Time of Seizure:** ___________
- **Duration:** ___________ (e.g., seconds/minutes)
- **Type of Seizure:** ___________ (e.g., focal, generalized, etc.)
- **Triggers (if known):** ___________ (e.g., stress, sleep, flashing lights)
- **Warning Signs (Aura):** ___________ (e.g., dizziness, visual changes)
- **Description:**

What Happened:

After Effects:

Medication Taken (before/after):

Notes:

WEEK 2 REVIEW
Week Starting: _____________

- **Number of Seizures:** _____________

Patterns Noticed:

Common Triggers:

- **Medication Adherence: Yes / No**

Side Effects:

Notes for Healthcare Provider:

Day 15

- **Date:** ____________
- **Time of Seizure:** ____________
- **Duration:** ____________ (e.g., seconds/minutes)
- **Type of Seizure:** ____________ (e.g., focal, generalized, etc.)
- **Triggers (if known):** ____________ (e.g., stress, sleep, flashing lights)
- **Warning Signs (Aura):** ____________ (e.g., dizziness, visual changes)
- **Description:**

What Happened:

After Effects:

Medication Taken (before/after):

Notes:

Day 16

- **Date:** ___________
- **Time of Seizure:** ___________
- **Duration:** ___________ (e.g., seconds/minutes)
- **Type of Seizure:** ___________ (e.g., focal, generalized, etc.)
- **Triggers (if known):** ___________ (e.g., stress, sleep, flashing lights)
- **Warning Signs (Aura):** ___________ (e.g., dizziness, visual changes)
- **Description:**

What Happened:

After Effects:

Medication Taken (before/after):

Notes:

Day 17

- **Date:** ___________
- **Time of Seizure:** ___________
- **Duration:** ___________ (e.g., seconds/minutes)
- **Type of Seizure:** ___________ (e.g., focal, generalized, etc.)
- **Triggers (if known):** ___________ (e.g., stress, sleep, flashing lights)
- **Warning Signs (Aura):** ___________ (e.g., dizziness, visual changes)
- **Description:**

What Happened:

After Effects:

Medication Taken (before/after):

**Notes:

Day 18

- **Date:** ___________
- **Time of Seizure:** ___________
- **Duration:** ___________ (e.g., seconds/minutes)
- **Type of Seizure:** ___________ (e.g., focal, generalized, etc.)
- **Triggers (if known):** ___________ (e.g., stress, sleep, flashing lights)
- **Warning Signs (Aura):** ___________ (e.g., dizziness, visual changes)
- **Description:**

What Happened:

After Effects:

Medication Taken (before/after):

Notes:

Day 19

- **Date:** ___________
- **Time of Seizure:** ___________
- **Duration:** ___________ (e.g., seconds/minutes)
- **Type of Seizure:** ___________ (e.g., focal, generalized, etc.)
- **Triggers (if known):** ___________ (e.g., stress, sleep, flashing lights)
- **Warning Signs (Aura):** ___________ (e.g., dizziness, visual changes)
- **Description:**

What Happened:

After Effects:

Medication Taken (before/after):

Notes:

Day 20

- **Date:** ___________
- **Time of Seizure:** ___________
- **Duration:** ___________ (e.g., seconds/minutes)
- **Type of Seizure:** ___________ (e.g., focal, generalized, etc.)
- **Triggers (if known):** ___________ (e.g., stress, sleep, flashing lights)
- **Warning Signs (Aura):** ___________ (e.g., dizziness, visual changes)
- **Description:**

What Happened:

After Effects:

Medication Taken (before/after):

Notes:

Day 21

- **Date:** ____________
- **Time of Seizure:** ____________
- **Duration:** ____________ (e.g., seconds/minutes)
- **Type of Seizure:** ____________ (e.g., focal, generalized, etc.)
- **Triggers (if known):** ____________ (e.g., stress, sleep, flashing lights)
- **Warning Signs (Aura):** ____________ (e.g., dizziness, visual changes)
- **Description:**

What Happened:

After Effects:

Medication Taken (before/after):

Notes:

WEEK 3 REVIEW

Week Starting: ______________

- **Number of Seizures:** ______________

Patterns Noticed:

Common Triggers:

- **Medication Adherence: Yes / No**

Side Effects:

Notes for Healthcare Provider:

Day 22

- **Date:** ___________
- **Time of Seizure:** ___________
- **Duration:** ___________ (e.g., seconds/minutes)
- **Type of Seizure:** ___________ (e.g., focal, generalized, etc.)
- **Triggers (if known):** ___________ (e.g., stress, sleep, flashing lights)
- **Warning Signs (Aura):** ___________ (e.g., dizziness, visual changes)
- **Description:**

What Happened:

After Effects:

Medication Taken (before/after):

Notes:

Day 23

- **Date:** ____________
- **Time of Seizure:** ____________
- **Duration:** ____________ (e.g., seconds/minutes)
- **Type of Seizure:** ____________ (e.g., focal, generalized, etc.)
- **Triggers (if known):** ____________ (e.g., stress, sleep, flashing lights)
- **Warning Signs (Aura):** ____________ (e.g., dizziness, visual changes)
- **Description:**

What Happened:

After Effects:

Medication Taken (before/after):

Notes:

Day 24

- **Date:** ___________
- **Time of Seizure:** ___________
- **Duration:** ___________ (e.g., seconds/minutes)
- **Type of Seizure:** ___________ (e.g., focal, generalized, etc.)
- **Triggers (if known):** ___________ (e.g., stress, sleep, flashing lights)
- **Warning Signs (Aura):** ___________ (e.g., dizziness, visual changes)
- **Description:**

What Happened:

After Effects:

Medication Taken (before/after):

Notes:

Day 25

- **Date:** ___________
- **Time of Seizure:** ___________
- **Duration:** ___________ (e.g., seconds/minutes)
- **Type of Seizure:** ___________ (e.g., focal, generalized, etc.)
- **Triggers (if known):** ___________ (e.g., stress, sleep, flashing lights)
- **Warning Signs (Aura):** ___________ (e.g., dizziness, visual changes)
- **Description:**

What Happened:

After Effects:

Medication Taken (before/after):

Notes:

Day 26

- **Date:** ____________
- **Time of Seizure:** ____________
- **Duration:** ____________ (e.g., seconds/minutes)
- **Type of Seizure:** ____________ (e.g., focal, generalized, etc.)
- **Triggers (if known):** ____________ (e.g., stress, sleep, flashing lights)
- **Warning Signs (Aura):** ____________ (e.g., dizziness, visual changes)
- **Description:**

What Happened:

After Effects:

Medication Taken (before/after):

Notes:

Day 27

- **Date:** ___________
- **Time of Seizure:** ___________
- **Duration:** ___________ (e.g., seconds/minutes)
- **Type of Seizure:** ___________ (e.g., focal, generalized, etc.)
- **Triggers (if known):** ___________ (e.g., stress, sleep, flashing lights)
- **Warning Signs (Aura):** ___________ (e.g., dizziness, visual changes)
- **Description:**

What Happened:

After Effects:

Medication Taken (before/after):

Notes:

Day 28

- **Date:** ___________
- **Time of Seizure:** ___________
- **Duration:** ___________ (e.g., seconds/minutes)
- **Type of Seizure:** ___________ (e.g., focal, generalized, etc.)
- **Triggers (if known):** ___________ (e.g., stress, sleep, flashing lights)
- **Warning Signs (Aura):** ___________ (e.g., dizziness, visual changes)
- **Description:**

What Happened:

After Effects:

Medication Taken (before/after):

Notes:

<u>WEEK 4 REVIEW</u>
Week Starting: ______________

• **Number of Seizures:** ______________

Patterns Noticed:

Common Triggers:

• **Medication Adherence: Yes / No**

Side Effects:

Notes for Healthcare Provider:

Day 29

- **Date:** ___________
- **Time of Seizure:** ___________
- **Duration:** ___________ (e.g., seconds/minutes)
- **Type of Seizure:** ___________ (e.g., focal, generalized, etc.)
- **Triggers (if known):** ___________ (e.g., stress, sleep, flashing lights)
- **Warning Signs (Aura):** ___________ (e.g., dizziness, visual changes)
- **Description:**

What Happened:

After Effects:

Medication Taken (before/after):

Notes:

Day 30

- **Date:** ___________
- **Time of Seizure:** ___________
- **Duration:** ___________ (e.g., seconds/minutes)
- **Type of Seizure:** ___________ (e.g., focal, generalized, etc.)
- **Triggers (if known):** ___________ (e.g., stress, sleep, flashing lights)
- **Warning Signs (Aura):** ___________ (e.g., dizziness, visual changes)
- **Description:**

What Happened:

After Effects:

Medication Taken (before/after):

Notes:

Day 31

- **Date:** ___________
- **Time of Seizure:** ___________
- **Duration:** ___________ (e.g., seconds/minutes)
- **Type of Seizure:** ___________ (e.g., focal, generalized, etc.)
- **Triggers (if known):** ___________ (e.g., stress, sleep, flashing lights)
- **Warning Signs (Aura):** ___________ (e.g., dizziness, visual changes)
- **Description:**

What Happened:

After Effects:

Medication Taken (before/after):

Notes:

Month Review

- **Month:** ___________
- **Total Seizures:** ___________

Most Common Triggers:

- **Most Common Time of Day:** ___________
- **Medication Review:**

Changes: Yes / No
Effectiveness:

Overall Patterns or Concerns:

Questions for Next Doctor's Appointment:

<u>Message from the Author:</u>

I hope you enjoyed this book, I love astrology and knew there was not a book such as this out on the shelf. I love metaphysical items as well. Please check out my other books:

-Life of Government Benefits

-My life of Hell

-My life with Hydrocephalus

-Red Sky

-World Domination:Woman's rule

-World Domination:Woman's Rule 2: The War

-Life and Banishment of Apophis: book 1

-The Kidney Friendly Diet

-The Ultimate Hemp Cookbook

-Creating a Dispensary(legally)

-Cleanliness throughout life: the importance of showering from childhood to adulthood.

-Strong Roots: The Risks of Overcoddling children

-Hemp Horoscopes: Cosmic Insights and Earthly Healing

- Celestial Hemp Navigating the Zodiac: Through the Green Cosmos

-Astrological Hemp: Aligning The Stars with Earth's Ancient Herb

-The Astrological Guide to Hemp: Stars, Signs, and Sacred Leaves

-Green Growth: Innovative Marketing Strategies for your Hemp Products and Dispensary

-Cosmic Cannabis

-Astrological Munchies

-Henry The Hemp

-Zodiacal Roots: The Astrological Soul Of Hemp

- Green Constellations: Intersection of Hemp and Zodiac

-Hemp in The Houses: An astrological Adventure Through The Cannabis Galaxy

-Galactic Ganja Guide

Heavenly Hemp
Zodiac Leaves
Doctor Who Astrology
Cannastrology
Stellar Satvias and Cosmic Indicas
<u>Celestial Cannabis: A Zodiac Journey</u>
AstroHerbology: The Sky and The Soil: Volume 1
AstroHerbology:Celestial Cannabis:Volume 2
Cosmic Cannabis Cultivation
The Starry Guide to Herbal Harmony: Volume 1
The Starry Guide to Herbal Harmony: Cannabis Universe: Volume 2

Yugioh Astrology: Astrological Guide to Deck, Duels and more
Nightmare Mansion: Echoes of The Abyss
Nightmare Mansion 2: Legacy of Shadows
Nightmare Mansion 3: Shadows of the Forgotten
Nightmare Mansion 4: Echoes of the Damned
The Life and Banishment of Apophis: Book 2
Nightmare Mansion: Halls of Despair
<u>Healing with Herb: Cannabis and Hydrocephalus</u>
<u>Planetary Pot: Aligning with Astrological Herbs: Volume 1</u>
Fast Track to Freedom: 30 Days to Financial Independence Using AI, Assets, and Agile Hustles
<u>Cosmic Hemp Pathways</u>
How to Become Financially Free in 30 Days: 10,000 Paths to Prosperity
Zodiacal Herbage: Astrological Insights: Volume 1
Nightmare Mansion: Whispers in the Walls
The Daleks Invade Atlantis
Henry the hemp and Hydrocephalus

10X The Kidney Friendly Diet
Cannabis Universe: Adult coloring book

Hemp Astrology: The Healing Power of the Stars

Zodiacal Herbage: Astrological Insights: Cannabis Universe: Volume 2

Planetary Pot: Aligning with Astrological Herbs: Cannabis Universes: Volume 2

Doctor Who Meets the Replicators and SG-1: The Ultimate Battle for Survival

Nightmare Mansion: Curse of the Blood Moon

The Celestial Stoner: A Guide to the Zodiac

Cosmic Pleasures: Sex Toy Astrology for Every Sign

Hydrocephalus Astrology: Navigating the Stars and Healing Waters

Lapis and the Mischievous Chocolate Bar

Celestial Positions: Sexual Astrology for Every Sign

Apophis's Shadow Work Journal: : A Journey of Self-Discovery and Healing

Kinky Cosmos: Sexual Kink Astrology for Every Sign

Digital Cosmos: The Astrological Digimon Compendium

Stellar Seeds: The Cosmic Guide to Growing with Astrology

Apophis's Daily Gratitude Journal

Cat Astrology: Feline Mysteries of the Cosmos

The Cosmic Kama Sutra: An Astrological Guide to Sexual Positions

Unleash Your Potential: A Guided Journal Powered by AI Insights

Whispers of the Enchanted Grove

Cosmic Pleasures: An Astrological Guide to Sexual Kinks

369, 12 Manifestation Journal

Whisper of the nocturne journal(blank journal for writing or drawing)

The Boogey Book
Locked In Reflection: A Chastity Journey Through Locktober
Generating Wealth Quickly:
How to Generate $100,000 in 24 Hours
Star Magic: Harness the Power of the Universe
The Flatulence Chronicles: A Fart Journal for Self-Discovery
The Doctor and The Death Moth

If you want solar for your home go here: https://www.harborso-
lar.live/apophisenterprises/

Get Some Tarot cards: https://www.makeplayingcards.com/sell/apophis-occult-shop

<u>**Get some shirts: https://www.bonfire.com/store/apophis-shirt-emporium/**</u>

Instagrams:
@apophis_enterprises,
@apophisbookemporium,
@apophisscardshop
Twitter: @apophisenterpr1
 Tiktok:@apophisenterprise
Youtube: @sg1fan23477, @FiresideRetreatKingdom

Podcast: Apophis Chat Zone: https://open.spotify.com/show/
5zXbrCLEV2xzCp8ybrfHsk?si=fb4d4fdbdce44dec

Newsletter: https://apophiss-newsletter-27c897.beehiiv.com/